Pharmacognosy and Phytochemistry Practical manual

Dr. G. Sumalatha

M.Pharm, Ph.D

Associate Professor

Department of Pharmacognosy

GBN Institute of Pharmacy

RangaReddy-501301,

Telangana State

India

Copyright

All rights reserved. No part of this book may be reproduced or transmitted in any form or by any means, electronic or mechanical including photocopying, recording, or any information storage and retrieval system without the prior written permission from the publisher and the copyright holder.

Copyright © 2017-Dr. G.Sumalatha
All rights reserved.
ISBN-13: **978-1979763608**
ISBN- 10: 1979763607

Contents

1. Introduction to Pharmacognosy
2. Morphological Analysis
3. Extracts
4. Compound Microscope
5. Microscopical Analysis
6. General qualitative chemical tests
7. Carbohydrates
8. Quantitative Secondary Phytochemical Estimation
9. Extraction of caffeine from tea powder
10. Extraction of lycopene from tomatoes
11. Isolation of Piperine from black pepper
12. Extraction of Essential Oils from Cinnamon, Clove and *Nigella sativa* by Distillation
13. Extraction of pectin from orange peel and lemon peel
14. Isolation of Berberine from *Berberis aristata*
15. Extraction of Nicotine from Cigarettes
16. Extraction of *Lawsonia inermis*
17. Isolation of Hesperidin from Orange Peel Using Soxhlet Extractor
18. Identification of Plant Pigments (Carotenoids) by Thin Layer Chromatography

19. TLC Analysis of Curcumin and its Derivatives of Turmeric

20. Thin Layer Chromatography (TLC) of flavonoid drugs

21. Thin Layer Chromatography (TLC) of Anthocyanins and Crocin

22. Identification of Anthraquinone Glycosides from Plant Extract

1. Introduction to Pharmacognosy

Pharmacognosy is the study of those natural substances, principally plants that find use in medicine. Pharmacognosy is closely related to both botany and plant chemistry of which both have been originated from the earlier scientific studies on medicinal plants.

Pharmacognosy is "the study of the physical, chemical, biochemical and biological properties of drugs, drug substances or potential drugs or drug substances of natural origin as well as the search for new drugs from natural sources.

2. Morphological Analysis

Morphological (=macroscopical) analysis is easy method for identifying crude drugs. Crude drugs are the dried, unprepared material of plant or animal origin. Most of the crude drugs are plant based. Plant form ranges from unicellular plants to the strongly differentiated higher plants. Characteristically the higher plants consist in the vegetative phase of roots, stems and leaves with flowers, fruits and seeds forming stages in the reproductive cycle. Some of the drugs are exudates (gums, resins) or they have been obtained by a secondary process (essential oils, fixed oils etc.). Due to the lack of modern analysis methods, the quality of crude drugs were based on the five senses (e.g., colour, odour, taste, shape, size, dimensions, surface characters, fracture and texture). With another words, morphological characters of crude drugs have been used for the quality assurance, authentication, and identification of adulteration.

It is important to interpret morphological and anatomical descriptions of crude drugs as found in pharmacopoeias and allied works and also to record adequately the features of whole or powdered drugs and adulterants of commercial significance.

Nomenclature:

The pharmaceutical names generally consist of two words. One of these is related to the scientific name of the plant from which the drug derives while the second indicates the plant part (bark, leaf etc.) used. The following terms are used to indicate the parts of plants:

Radix = root: The term does not completely coincide with the botanical concept. A drug termed a radix may sometimes also contain rhizomes.

Rhizoma = rhizome; A subterranean stem, generally carrying lateral roots.

Tuber: A nutritious subterranean organ, which, in a botanical sense, is a rhizome. A tuber is a thick organ, mainly consisting of parenchymatous storage tissue (generally containing starch) and a small proportion of lignified elements.

Bulbus = onion: Botanically, an onion is a stem, surrounded by thick nutritious leaves that are usually low in chlorophyll content.

Lignum = wood: Drugs for which this term is used are obtained from plants with secondary thickening and consist of the woody parts of the xylem.

Cortex = bark: Barks are obtained from plants with secondary thickening and, unlike the botanical definition of the term, they consist of all the tissues outside the cambium. Such drugs can be collected from roots, stems and branches.

Folium = leaf: Leaf consists of the middle leaves of the plant.

Flos = flower: The crude drug may consist of single flowers and/or entire inflorescences.

Fructus = fruit: The pharmacognostical term is not always synonymous with the botanical one. Thus, the drug drug Cynosbati fructus cum semen (rose hips) is, botanically speaking, a swollen receptacle carrying the true fruits (nuts). Also the second part of the term - semen - is thus not correct from a botanical standpoint as semen is the pharmaceutical term for seed (see below). There is also another crude drug consisting only of the receptacle without fruits. The pharmaceutical name for this crude drug is Cynosbati fructus sine semen.

Pericarpium = fruit peel or pericarp which is the common botanical term.

Semen = seed: The drug can consist either of the seed, as removed from the fruit, or of a part of the seed, as in Colae semen, which does not contain the testa or seed coat.

Herba = herb: The crude drug consists of the aerial parts of the plant; thus, stems as well as leaves, flowers and fruits, if any, are included.

Aetherolum = essential or volatile oil is, a product obtained from plant material. It usually possesses a distinctive odour and consists of a complex mixture of comparatively volatile components.

Oleum = oil, is a fixed oil prepared from plant material by pressing.

Pyroleum = tar, is prepared by dry distillation of plant material.

Resina = resin, is obtained either from secretory structures in certain plants or by distillation of a balsam (see below). In the latter case, it is the residue after distillation. Balsamum = balsam, is a solution of resin in a volatile oil and is generally produced by special cells in the plant.

3. Extracts

Extracts can be defined as preparations of crude drugs which contain all the constituents which are soluble in the solvent used in making the extract.

In dry extracts (extracta sicca) all solvent has been removed. Soft extracts (extracta spissa) and fluid extracts (extracta fluida) are prepared with mixtures of water and ethanol as solvent. A soft extract contains 15-25 % residual water. A fluid extract is concentrated to such an extent that the soluble constituents of one part of the crude drug are contained in one or two parts of the extract. Tinctures are prepared by extraction of the crude drug with five to ten parts of ethanol of varying concentration, without concentration of the final product. For both extracts and tinctures the weight-ratio drug/extract should always be stated.

Thus if 100 g of a crude drug yields 20 g of dry extract the ratio is 5:1. Consequently, if the same amount of crude drug is used to prepare 1000 g of tincture, the ratio is 1:10. By definition the crude drug/extract ratio for a fluid extract is 1:1 or 1:2.

Choice of solvent:

The ideal solvent for a certain pharmacologically active constituent should:

1. Be highly selective for the compound to be extracted.
2. Have a high capacity for extraction in terms of coefficient of saturation of the compound in the medium.
3. Not react with the extracted compound or with other compounds in the plant material.
4. Have a low price.
5. Be harmless to man and to the environment.
6. Be completely volatile

Extraction procedures

Maceration, Percolation, Counter current extraction.

The ethanol is usually mixed with water to induce swelling of the plant particles and to increase the porosity of the cell walls which facilitates the diffusion of extracted substances from inside the cells to the surrounding solvent. For extraction of barks, roots, woody parts and seeds the ideal alcohol/water ratio is about 7:3 or 8:2. For leaves or aerial green parts the ratio 1:1 is usually preferred in order to avoid extraction of chlorophyll.

Maceration:

This is the simplest procedure for obtaining an extract and is suitable both for small quantities of drug and for industrial production. Simple maceration is performed at room temperature by mixing the ground drug with the solvent (drug/solvent ratio: 1:5 or 1:10) and leaving the mixture for several days with occasional shaking or stirring. The extract is then separated from the plant particles by straining. The procedure is repeated once or twice with fresh solvent.

Finally the last residue of extract is pressed out of the plant particles using a mechanical press or a centrifuge.

Percolation:

Simple percolation is a procedure in which the plant material is packed in a tube-like percolator which is fitted with a filter sieve at the bottom. Fresh solvent is fed from the top until the extract recovered at the bottom of the tube does not contain any solute. This is a slow and costly process requiring large quantities of fresh solvent.

A technical problem in percolation is to ensure an equal How of solvent through the mass of crude drug powder. The drug should not be too finely ground to allow a reasonably fast passage of the solvent. A particle size of 1-3 mm is usually sufficient. Before the material is loaded into the percolator it should be moistened with the solvent and allowed to swell. It is then carefully packed into the percolator in such a way that the layer formed is as uniform as possible. Solvent is administered at the top and passes through the drug. The extract is collected at the bottom or is passed on to the next percolator if a battery is used. Transport of solvent can be achieved by gravity or by pumping.

Counter current extraction:

This is a continuous process in which the plant material moves against the solvent. Several types of extractors are available. In the screw extractor the plant material is transported by a screw through a tube and meets the solvent which is pumped in the opposite direction.

Extraction with supercritical fluids:

At a sufficiently low temperature a gas may be made to liquefy by applying pressure to reduce the volume. However, there is a temperature above which it is impossible to liquefy the gas no matter how great a pressure is applied. This temperature is called the critical temperature. The minimum pressure necessary to bring about liquefaction at the critical temperature is called the critical pressure. The combination of critical pressure and critical temperature is characteristic of the particular substance and is called the critical point. Gases at temperatures and pressures above the critical point are called supercritical gases or supercritical fluids. Only gases which can be converted into the supercritical state at attainable pressures and temperatures can be considered for extraction use.

Critical temperatures and pressures		
Fluid	Critical temp., °C	Critical pressure, bar
Ethylene	9.3	50.4
Carbon dioxide	31.1	73.8
Ethane	32.3	48.8
Nitrous oxide	36.5	72.7
Propylene	91.9	46.2
Propane	96.7	42.5
Ammonia	132.5	112.8
Hexane	234.2	30.3
Water	374.2	220.5

Purification and concentration of extracts:

The methods used are decantation, centrifugation and filtration. For the manufacture of fluid and soft extracts the clarified extract must be concentrated. Preparation of a dry extract requires complete removal of the solvent. Concentration is a tricky stage in the process in which many chemically labile compounds may undergo degradation, mainly due to the temperature. Concentration in vacuo is therefore the preferred method by which the extract can be kept at 25-30°C during the whole procedure. Several types of concentrators are available.

Drying of extracts:

The concentrators (rotary evaporator) can be used for production of fluid and soft extracts but are not suitable for complete drying of an extract.

Drying in cabinet driers: Hot air (60–80 °C) is blown over the shelves.

Drying in atomizers (spray drying) is suitable for industrial production.

Freeze-drying: Freeze-drying (lyophilization) is a very mild method. Frozen material is placed in an evacuated apparatus which has a cold surface maintained at -60 to -80°C. Water vapour from the frozen material then passes rapidly to the cold surface.

4. Compound Microscope:

The Compound microscope is composed of both mechanical and optical units and essentially consists of the following parts:

1. A lens system
2. Provision for focusing the lens system
3. Stage
4. Device for providing satisfactory illumination

A lens system consists of two lenses: the objective and eyepiece (ocular). These are separated and held in correct relative position by the body tube, the eye piece being fitted into the upper end and the objective screwed to the lower end. Together, they form the combined optical unit, which is fixed to a stand on which it can be raised or lowered by means of coarse and fine adjustments, so that the optical point is focused on the slide which is being examined.

The objective lens enlarges the object and projects its image in the direction of the ocular lens.

In order to provide different degrees of magnification, the microscope may be equipped with a revolving nose piece, which carries three or four objectives, and this may be attached to the lower end of the body tube.

The function of the eyepiece is to magnify further the image formed by the objective.

The coarse adjustment knob serves to focus the microscope on the specimen by raising or lowering the lens system.

The specimen to be examined is illuminated by another lens system, called the condenser. Underneath the stage is another optical unit, the substage condenser and attached to it is substage iris diaphragm. The condenser is used to focus light on the object and can be moved up and down by means of a milled head. The role of condenser is usually underestimated, because it does not contribute to magnification. However, its proper use influences the quality of the image observed. The diaphragm can be adjusted by means of a small lever to control the amount of light which reaches the field being viewed. A filter holder, in the form of a metal ring is often placed beneath the iris diaphragm. It can usually be swung out of position by a short projecting lever. Discs of coloured glass may be provided for use in the filter holder.

5. Microscopical Analysis

Aim of the microscopic analysis of the powdered crude drugs is also identification and authentication. The structure of cell wall, cell shape and cell contents are microscopical characters of the medicinal plants and they are of value in identification and in the detection of adulteration.

The aim of the microscopical examination of crude drugs:

i. The determination of the size, shape and relative positions of the different cell and tissues
ii. The determination of the chemical nature of the cell wall
iii. The determination of the form and chemical nature of the cell contents.

This method is useful for identifying herbal drug powders and for distinguishing species with similar morphological characters. By means of microscopic techniques, structural and cellular features of herbs are examined in order to determine their botanical origins and assess their qualities. These are:

1. The Cell Wall
   Cellulose walls, lignified walls, suberized and cutinized walls, mucilaginous cell walls, chitinous cell walls
2. Parenchymatous Tissue
3. The Epidermis
4. Epidermal Trichomes
5. The Endodermis
6. Cork Tissue
7. Collenchyma
8. Sclereids (Sclereid or Stone cells)
9. Xylem (Tracheids, vessels or trachea, xylem fibres, xylem paranchyma)
10. Phloem (Sieve tubes, companian cells, phloem paranchyma and secretory cells)
11. Secretory Tissues (Secretory cells, secretory cavities, canals and latex tissue).
12. Ergastic Cell Contents
    Starch, proteins, fixed oil, gums, mucilage, volatile oils, crystals

Different types of starches

Starch Drug : Potato starch Plant : *Solanum tuberosum* Family : Solanaceae	
Drug : Maize starch Plant : *Zea mays* Family : Graminae	
Drug : Rice starch Plant : *Oryza sativa* Family : Graminae	
Drug : Wheat starch Plant : *Triticum aestivum* Family : Graminae	

Different types of calcium oxalate crystals

Simple crystals Drug : Hyoscyami folium (Folia Hyoscyami) Plant : *Hyoscyamus niger*, Banotu Family : Solanaceae	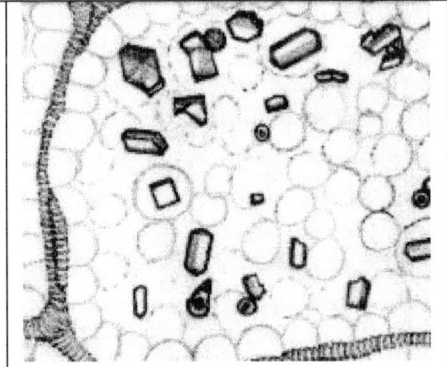
Crystal sand Drug : Cinchona cortex (Cortex Chinae) Plant : *Cinchona pubescens*, Kına kına Family : Rubiaceae	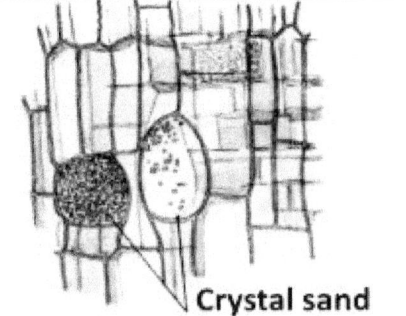
Druse crystals Drug : Rhei radix (Rhizoma Rhei) Plant : *Rheum palmatum*, Ravent Family : Polygonaceae	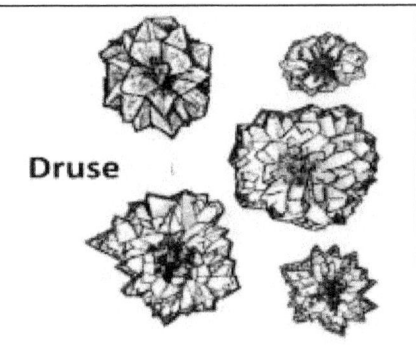

Raphide crystals Drug : Scillae bulbus (Bulbus Scillae) Plant : *Urginea maritima* Family : Liliacae (Alliaceae)	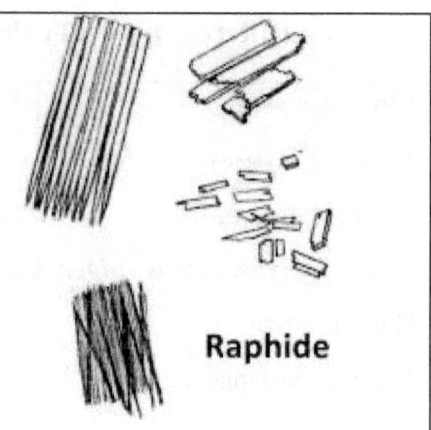

Non-glandular or covering trichomes

Multicellular trichomes Drug : Thymi folium Plant : *Thymus serpyllum*, Kekik Family : Lamiaceae	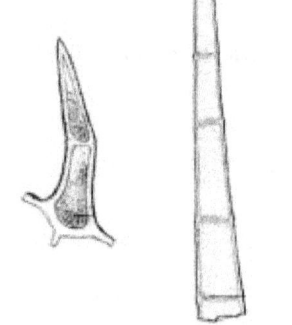
Unicellular trichomes Drug : Malva folium Plant : *Malva sylvestris*, Ebegümeci Family : Malvaceae	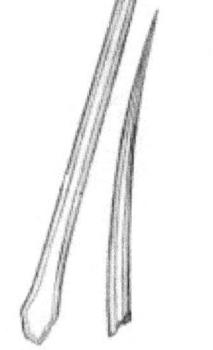

Unicellular trichomes Drug : Melissa folium Plant : *Melissa officinalis*, Oğulotu Family : Lamiaceae	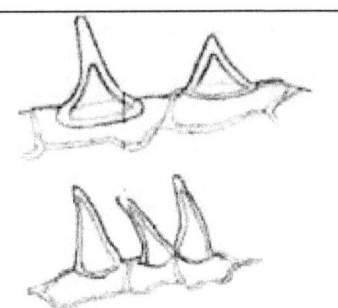
Stellate trichomes (Star shaped trichomes) Drug : Rosmarini folium Plant : *Rosmarinus officinalis*, Biberiye Family : Lamiaceae	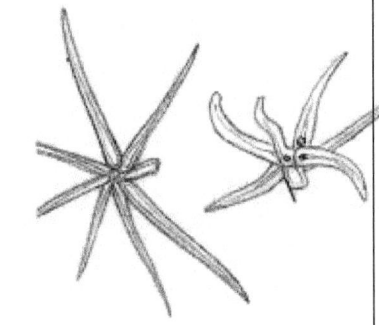
Stalked Stellate (star) trichomes Drug : Malvae sylvestris flos Plant : *Malva sylvestris*, Ebegümeci Family : Malvaceae	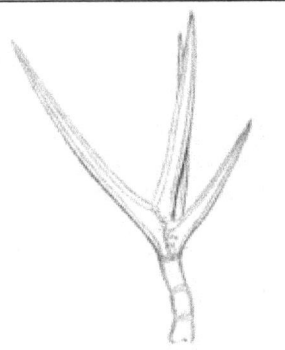

T-shaped trichomes Drug : Absinthi herba Plant : *Artemisia absinthium*, Pelin Otu Family : Asteraceae	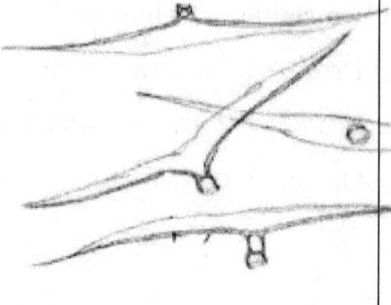
Branched trichomes Drug : Lavandulae flos Plant : *Lavandula angustifolia*, Lavanta Family : Lamiaceae	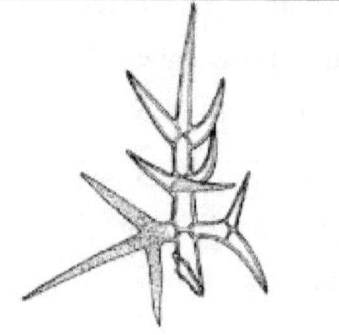

Different types of stomata

Anomocytic (irregular-celled, ranunculaceous) type: Stoma surrounded by a limited number of cells that are indistinguishable in size or form from those of the remainder of the epidermis. Eg: Digitalis	
Anisocytic (unequal-celled, cruciferous) type: Stoma surrounded by three cells of	

which one is distinctly smaller than the other two. Eg: Datura, Belladonna	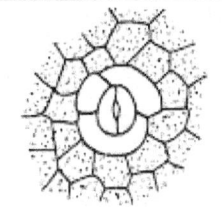
Paracytic (parallel-celled, rubiaceous) type: Stoma accompanied on either side by one or more subsidiary cells parallel to the long axis of the pore and guard cells. Eg: Coca, Senna	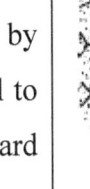
Diacytic (cross-celled, caryophyllaceous) type: Stoma enclosed by a pair of subsidiary cells whose common wall is at right angles to the guard cells. Eg: Vasaka, Spearmint	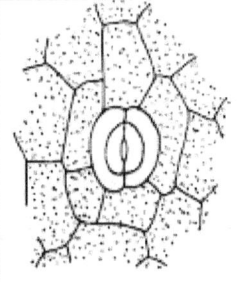
Actinocytic or radiate celled: Stoma is surrounded by four or more subsidiary cells, elongated radially to the stoma. Eg: Lannea	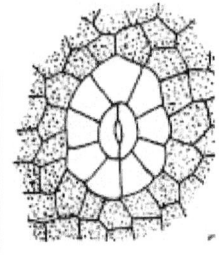

Cyclocytic type: a similar number of cells forms a narrow ring round each stoma' (a similar number = four or more). Eg: Schinopsis	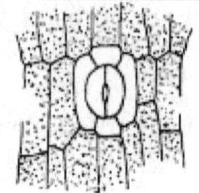
Tetracytic type: The guard cells are surrounded by four subsidiary cells, two lateral and two polar ones.	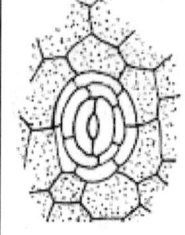

Secretory tissues

Glandular trichomes Drug : Mentha folium Plant : *Mentha piperita* Family : Lamiaceae (Labiatae)	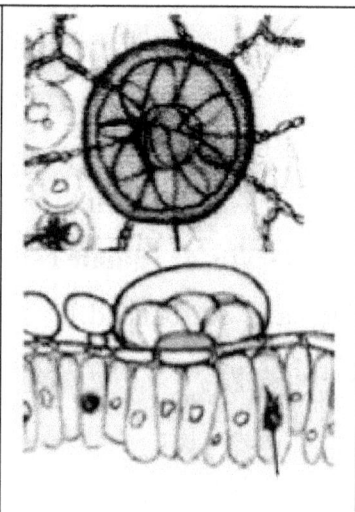

Schizogenous oil glands Drug : Eucalyptus folium Plant : *Eucalyptus globulus* Family : Myrtaceae	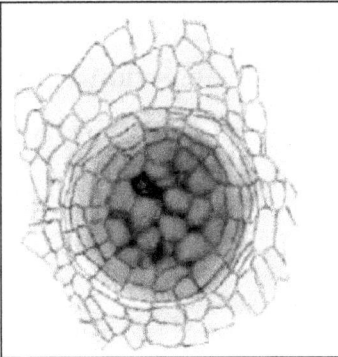
Secretory canals Drug : Anisi fructus Plant : *Pimpinella anisum* Family : Apiaceae (Umbelliferae)	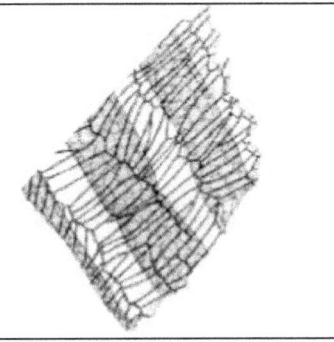

Glandular trichomes

Glandular trichome with unicellular stalk and multicellular head	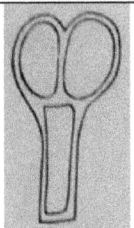
Uniseriate glandular trichome with unicellular head	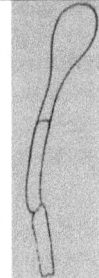

Multiseriate multicellular glandular trichome with multicellular head	
Multicellular glandular head with unicellular stalk	

Xylem vessels

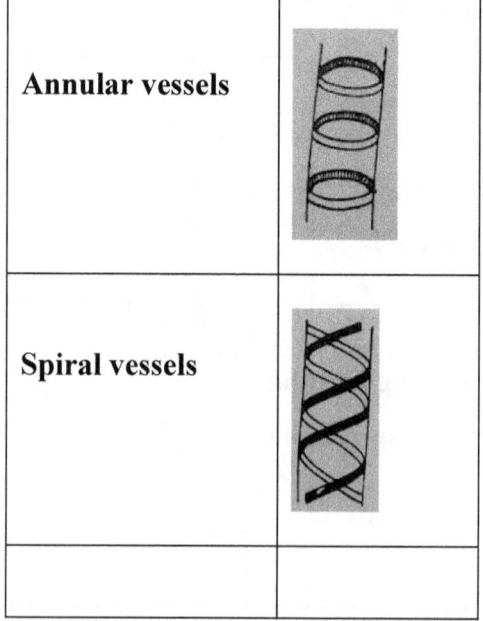

Annular vessels	
Spiral vessels	

Scalariform vessel	
Reticulate vessel	

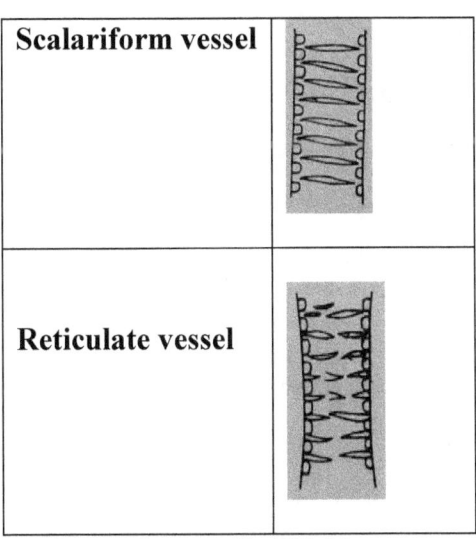

Sclereids: Schlerenchyma, Stone cells, Idioblasts

Sclereids Stone cells Drug : Cinnamomi cortex Plant : *Cinnamomum zeylanicum* Family : Lauraceae	
Sclereids Stone cells Drug : Caryophylli flos Plant : *Syzygium aromaticum*, Karanfil Family : Myrtaceae	

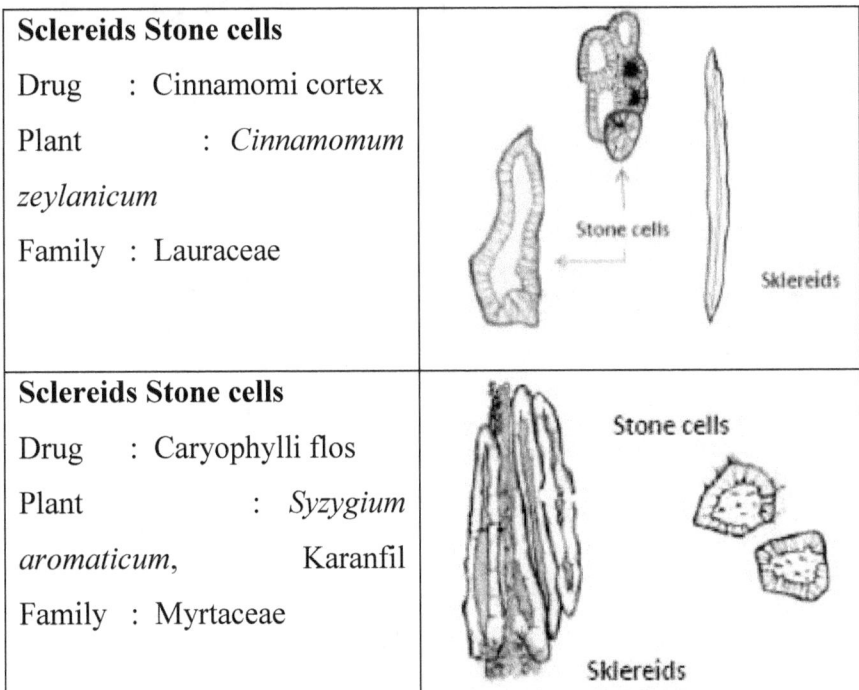

Sclereids Stone cells Drug : Gallae, Mazı Plant : *Quercus infectoria*, Meşe Family : Fagaceae	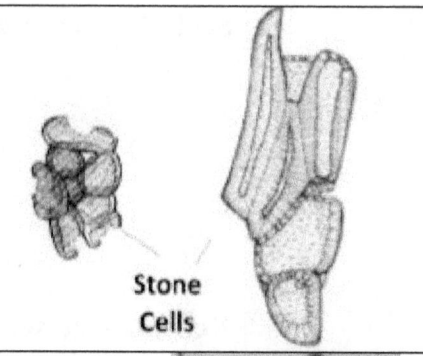
Sclereids Idioblast (Astrosclereids) Plant : Nuphar sp, Nymphaea sp. Family : Nymphaceae	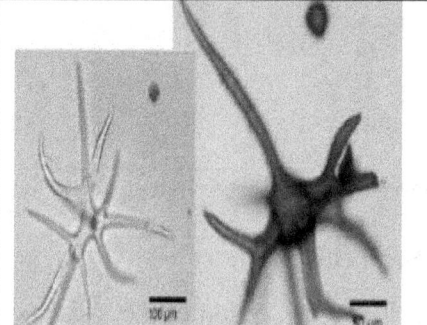

Pollens

Pollen Drug : Malvae folium, Malvae flos Plant : *Malva sylvestris*, Mallow Family : Malvaceae	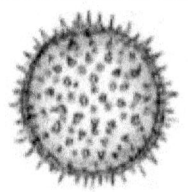
Pollen Drug : Lavandulae flos Plant : *Lavandula angustifolia*, Levander, Lavanta Family : Lamiaceae	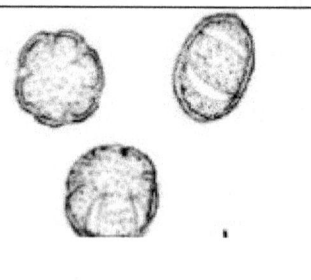

Pollen Drug : Helichrysi flos Plant : *Helichrysum arenarium*, Immortelle Family : Asteraceae	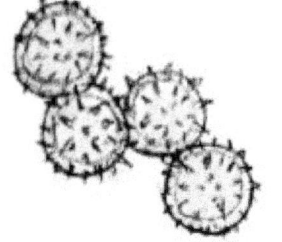
Pollen Drug : Croci stigma Plant : *Crocus sativus*, Saffron, Safran Family : Iridaceae	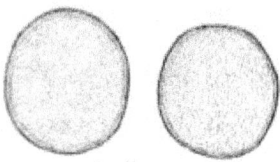

6. **General qualitative chemical tests:**

Test for Alkaloids

i) **Dragendorff's test:** Extract was treated with few drops of Dragendorff's reagent (potassium bismuth iodide solution). The reddish brown precipitate indicated the presence of Alkaloids.

ii) **Wagner's test:** Extract was treated with few drops of Wagner's reagent (iodine-potassium iodide solution). The reddish brown precipitate indicated the presence of Alkaloids.

iii) **Mayer's test:** Extract was treated with few drops of Mayer's reagent (potassium mercuric iodide solution). The white or pale precipitate indicated the presence of Alkaloids.

iv) **Hager's test:** Extract was treated with hager's reagent (picric acid), appearance of yellow colour precipitate indicated the presence of Alkaloids.

Test for Flavonoids

i) Shinoda test: Crude extracts was mixed with few fragments of magnesium ribbon and concentrated HCl was added drop wise. Appearance of pink scarlet colour after few minutes indicated the presence of flavonoids.

ii) Sodium hydroxide test: Few quantity of the each portion was dissolved in water and filtered; to this 2 ml of the 10% aqueous sodium hydroxide was later added to produce a yellow colouration. A change in colour from yellow to colourless on addition of dilute hydrochloric acid which indicated the presence of flavonoids.

iii) Zinc test: 2 ml extract was treated with Zinc dust and concentrated Hydrochloric acid, development of red colour indicated presence of Flavonoid

Test for Phenols

i) Ferric chloride test: Extract was treated with 2ml of water and 10% aqueous ferric chloride solution. Blue or green colour precipitate indicated presence of the phenol.

ii) Gelatin test: Ethanolic extract was added to about 1% solution of gelatin containing 10% sodium chloride. Formation of white precipitate indicated presence of the phenol.

Test for Saponins

i) Foam test: 5ml of filtrate was diluted with 20ml of water and vigorously shaken. The test tube was observed for the presence of stable foam upon standing.

Test for Steroids

Liebermann Burchard test: Concentrated extracts was added with 2ml of acetic anhydride and 1 ml of concentrated sulphuric acid development of colour bluish to green indicated the presence of steroids.

Test for Terpenoids

Salkowski test: 2 ml of each extracts was mixed with 2ml of chloroform and concentrated sulphuric acid (3ml) was carefully added to form a layer. An appearance of red colour indicated the presence of steroids

Test for Tannins

i) Ferric chloride test: The ethanolic extract is treated with 2 ml of Ferric chloride solution. The blue black precipitation is observed.

ii) Alkaline reagent test: Extract was treated with 10% sodium hydroxide solution formation of intense yellow colour indicated the presence of tannins.

iii) Gelatin test: Extract was treated with aqueous solution of gelatin and added sodium chloride, white buff colour precipitate indicated the presence of tannins.

Test for Cardiac glycosides

i). Keller-Killani test: Extracts was treated with 1ml of Ferric chloride reagent (mixture of 5% of Ferric chloride and 99 volume of glacial acetic acid). To this solution few drop of cons. Sulphuric acid was added appearance of greenish blue color within few minutes indicated the presence of cardiac glycosides.

ii). **Legal test:** Extracts was treated with few ml of pyridine add 2 drop of nitroprusside and 1 drop of 20% sodium hydroxide solution deep red colour indicated the presence of cardiac glycosides.

Specific Test for Alkaloids

Vitali's Test:

1. Evaporate 0.5 ml of alkaloid solution to dryness in a porcelain dish.
2. Add 2 drops of conc. Nitric acid.
3. Evaporate again on water bath to dryness (leaving a yellow residue)
4. Dissolve yellow residue with acetone.
5. Add a few drops of potassium hydroxide solution. (Formation of violet colour indicates a positive result)

Fluorescence Test:

1. In a test tube add 1 ml of alkaloid solution
2. Add 1 ml of dilute sulphuric acid.
3. Examine the test tube at 365 nm UV.
4. Formation of blue fluorescence under UV indicates positive result.

Murexide Test:

1. Evaporate 0.5 ml of alkaloid solution to dryness in a porcelain dish.
2. Add 0.5 ml of conc. Hydrochloric acid and 0.1 g Potassium chlorate. Take care of bubbling and fire
3. Evaporate to dryness over a water bath to form a yellow residue …Crimson color.

4. Add 2 drops of diluted ammonia (Purple colour indicates positive result)

Chen's Test:

1. In a test tube add 0.5 ml of the alkaloidal solution.
2. Add a few drops of diluted Hydrochloric acid.
3. Add 2 drops of 5% copper sulphate solution.
4. Add 1 ml of 20% sodium hydroxide and shake.
5. Watch for reddish-purple colour.
6. Add 1 ml of ether and shake.
7. Watch for the formation of the upper purple layer and the aqueous blue lower layer.

Detection of Cardiac Glycosides

Extraction:

Extract 5 g of powdered drug by boiling in a beaker for 5 min with 50 ml of 70 % alcohol and filter. Purification: Dilute the filtrate with equal volume of water and 1 ml of strong lead acetate solution and filter off the precipitate. Shake the filtrate with 50 ml of chloroform and take 18 ml of the chloroform extract after being dried on anhydrous sodium sulphate. Divide into four equal portions and evaporate off the solvent in porcelain dish using water bath under fume cupboard.

I. Test for the Butenolide Ring:

a. Kedde's test: Re-dissolve one portion of the residue in 2 ml of freshly prepared 3, 5-dinitrobenzoic acid solution (0.1 g of 3, 5-dinitrobenzoic acid dissolved in 10 ml methanol) and add 1 ml of 1 N sodium hydroxide solution. Allow standing for a few minutes and observe the change in colour and record the time required for colour development.

b. Baljet test: Re-dissolve the second portion of the residue in 5 ml methanol and add equivalent volume of freshly prepared Baljet's reagent (9.5 ml of 1% picric acid mixed with 0.5 ml of 10% sodium hydroxide). Allow standing for a few minutes. Observe the change in colour and record the time required for colour developments.

c. Legal's test: Re-dissolve the third portion of the residue in pyridine and add few drops of 2% sodium nitroprusside with few drops of 20% sodium hydroxide. Allow standing for a few minutes, and observe the change in colour and record the time required for colour development.

II. Test for deoxy sugars:

a. Keller-Kiliani test: Re-dissolve the forth portion of the residue in 3 ml glacial acetic acid containing 2 drops of ferric chloride solution, stir and pour the solution carefully into a dry test tube containing 2 ml of conc. sulphuric acid so that a two-phase system is produced. Observe the colour developed immediately at the interphase, record the change in the colour of the upper phase which will take place and the time required.

b. Xanthydrol-HCl test: Re-dissolve the fifth portion of the residue in 3 ml Xanthydrol-HCl (100 ml 96% acetic acid and 10 ml 37% conc. Hydrochloric acid mixed with 0.1 ml of 10% Xanthydrol solution.). Heat the mixture for 3 minutes in water bath. Allow standing for a few minute observe the change in the colour and record the time required for the colour development.

III. Test for the steroidal nucleus: Re-dissolve the last portion of the residue in 2 ml acetic anhydride and cool with ice. Add carefully 1 drop of conc. sulphuric acid (Liebermann- Burchard's test) allow standing for a few minutes, observe the change in the colour and record the time required for the colour development.

7. **Carbohydrates**

<u>**Starch**</u>

<u>**Definition:**</u>

Carbohydrates: natural plant products – organic compounds consist of C, H and O.

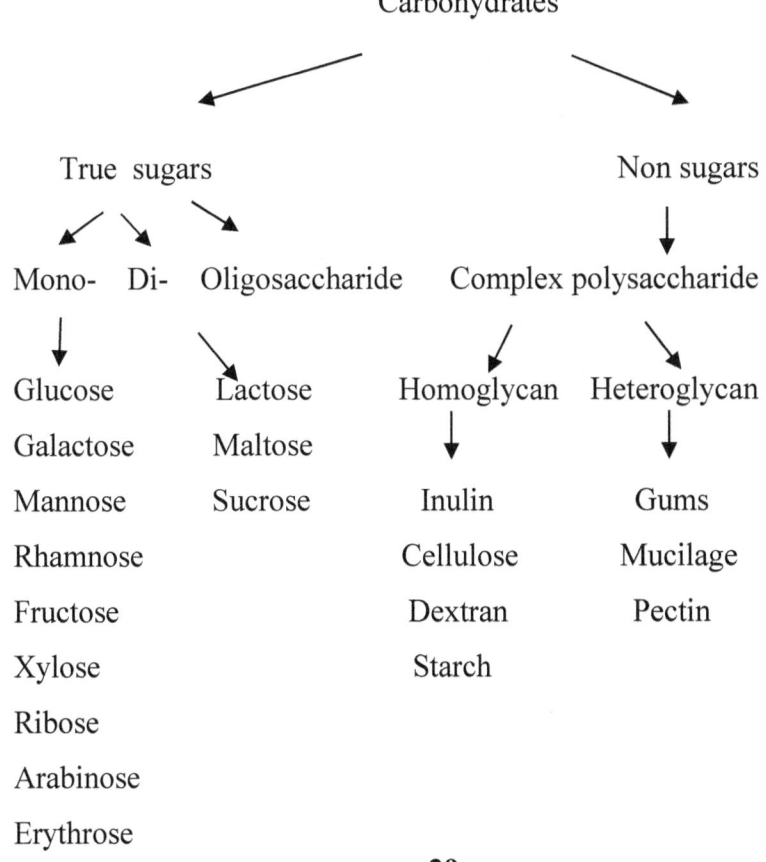

Complex polysaccharides: substances with very high molecular weight and consist of a large number of monosaccharide units linked together through glycosidic linkage.

Starch (Amylum):

Natural plant product which is a mixture of amylose (25%) and amylopectin (75%).

Amylose:
- Linear molecule consists of 250 – 300 units of α – D – glucose units linked together through α – 1,4 glycosidic linkage.
- More water soluble than amylopectin
- Amylose + I_2 → blue color

Amylopectin:
- Branched molecule consists of more than 1000 units of α- D – glucose linked together through α – 1,4 and α- 1,6 glycosidic linkage.
- Amylopectin is less water soluble than amylose.
- Amylopectin + I_2 → violet color

Plants containing starch:
- ✓ Cereal seeds contain 50- 65 % starch
- ✓ Ginger rhizomes 50% starch.
- ✓ Potato tubers 80- 90% starch.

Commercial sources of starch:

1. Corn starch: isolated from the caryopses of *Zea mays L.* – (*Graminae*)
2. Wheat starch: isolated from the caryopses of *Triticum aestivum L.* – (*Graminae*)
3. Rice starch: isolated from the caryopses of *Oryza sativa L.* – (*Graminae*)
4. Potato starch: isolated from the tubers of *Solanum tuberosum L.* – (*Solanaceae*)

Properties of Starch:

1. White mass powder, odorless with starchy taste
2. Insoluble in water and form colloidal solution with water.
3. Starch + I_2 → Deep blue color.
4. Starch + NaOH or chloral hydrate → gelatinization
5. Starch + H_2O → gel (with heat)
6. Corn starch and wheat starch have neutral pH

Rice starch has slightly alkaline pH.

Potato starch has slightly acidic pH.

Identification tests for starch:

1) Give positive reaction with Fehling's solution test:

   Starch + HCl (hydrolysis) + NaOH (neutralization) + Fehling's solution → Red colour

2) Give positive reaction with Molisch's test

   Starch + H_2SO_4 + α- naphthol → Purple ring

3) Starch + H_2O → gel (jelly form) with heat

4) Starch + $I_2 \rightarrow$ deep blue $\rightarrow$ colour disappears (with heating) $\rightarrow$ the colour reappears with cooling.

The general uses:
1. Nutritive.
2. Demulcent.
3. Pharmaceutical uses as tablets filler and binder.
4. Antipruritic: Baby paste®-(Vitamed company) used in case of diaper rash, skin irritation (ZnO, Starch).
5. Industrial uses: papers, clothes.
6. Antidote in case of poisoning from Iodine.

8. Quantitative Secondary Phytochemical Estimation

Total Alkaloid Estimation by using Harborn (1973)

Method 5g of sample was weighed separately into a 250 ml capacity beaker and added 200 ml of 10% solvent of acetic acid in ethanol then covered the beaker to check evaporations of solvent and allowed to stand for 4 hour. This was filtered and extracts was concentrated on water bath to ¼ of original volume then cons. ammonium hydroxide was added drop wise into concentrated extracts until the precipitation was completed. The solution was allowed to settle the precipitate and filtered. Filtered precipitate washed with dil. ammonium hydroxide and then again filtered. This precipitate residue is alkaloid which was dried and weighed.

Weight of total alkaloids: $(W_2-W_1)/W_3$ g,

% Yields of Alkaloid= $(W_2-W_1)/W_3 \times 100$

Where,

W_1 = weight of crucible,

W_2 = weight of crucible with alkaloids,

W_3 = initial weight of plant sample taken for estimation.

Total Flavonoids Estimation by Using Boham and Kocipai (1994) Method

10 g of powder sample was weighed into a 250 ml capacity beaker and added 100 ml of 80% aqueous methanol for extraction at room temperature. This was filtered through Whatman No. 42 (125 mm) filter paper and extracts was collected into another 250 ml capacity beaker. Extraction procedure repeated in same used sample separately and extract was recollected. Collected extract then transferred into crucible and evaporated till dryness on water bath and weighed.

Weight of total flavonoids: $(W_2-W_1)/W_3$ g,

% Yields of Flavonoids = $(W_2-W_1)/W_3 \times 100$

Where,

W_1 = weight of crucible,

W_2 = weight of crucible with flavonoids,

W_3 = initial weight of plant sample taken for estimation.

Total Saponin Estimation By Using Nahapetian and Bassiri (1975) Method

Suspension was prepared of 10 g of powder sample in 100 ml of 20% ethanol. This sample suspension was heated over water bath for 4 hour at 55°C with continuous stirring. This sample was filtered and extract was collected in 200 ml capacity of beaker. Obtained residue re- extracted with 100 ml of 20% ethanol. Combine extracts heated over water bath at about 90 till volume was reduced to 40 ml. The concentrate was transferred into a 250 ml separating funnel and 10 ml of diethyl ether was added and shaken vigorously. The aqueous layer was recovered while the ether layer was discarded. The purification process was repeated. 30 ml of n-butanol was added. The combine n- butanol extracts were washed twice with 10 ml of 5% aqueous sodium chloride. The remaining solution was heated in a water bath. After evaporation the sample were dried in the oven and weighted.

Weight of total saponins: $(W_2-W_1)/W_3$ g,

% Yields of Saponins= $(W_2-W_1)/W_3 \times 100$

Where,

W_1 = weight of crucible,

W_2 = weight of crucible with saponins,

W_3 = initial weight of plant sample taken for estimation.

Determination of total phenolic compound

Total phenol was determined by Folin–Ciocalteau reagent. A dilute extract or gallic acid was mixed with Folin–Ciocalteau reagent (5 ml, 1:10 diluted with distilled water) and aqueous 7.5% sodium carbonate solution (4 ml). The mixtures were allowed to stand for 15 minutes and the total phenols were determined at 765 nm. A standard curve was prepared using gallic acid. Total phenol values were expressed in terms of gallic acid used as a reference compound.

Determination of total tannins compound

A volume of 1 ml with duplicates of sample extract of concentrations (500 µg/ml) was pipetted out in test tubes. The volume was made up to 1 ml with distilled water, and 1 ml of water served as a blank. To this, 0.5 ml Folins-phenol reagent (1:2), followed by 5 ml of 35% sodium carbonate was added and kept at room temperature for 5 minutes. Blue color was formed. The color intensity was read at 640 nm. A standard graph of gallic acid was plotted, from which the tannin content of the extract was determined

9. Extraction of caffeine from tea powder

Procedure:
1. Weigh tea from 20 tea bags, 3 spoons Arabic coffee.
2. Add 100 ml of boiling distilled water and stir for 7 min.
3. Filter by filter paper- cool the filtrate in an ice bath.

Extraction:
4. Pour the cold tea filtrate into a separating funnel.
5. Slowly add 20 ml dichloromethane and gently stir the 2 layers for about 5 min.
6. Replace the Separating funnel into the stand, remove the stopper and allow separating for about 5 min.
7. Collect the organic phase into conical flask (Don't allow any of the darker material to escape through the stopcock).
8. Repeat the extraction twice more with fresh 20 ml of dichloromethane.

9. Add these 2 dichloromethane layers to the first (If an emulsion remains in the dichloromethane, filter through a Buchner funnel).
10. Return the organic phase to the SF and extract with 20 ml 6M sodium hydroxide (twice) and once with 20 ml distilled water.
11. Collect the dichloromethane layer into conical flask.
12. Dry the solution by adding 1 teaspoonful of anhydrous Magnesium sulphate, and then allow standing 5 min.
13. Filter and weigh empty flask.
14. Transfer the filtrate into flask and evaporate dichloromethane on the water bath.
15. Weigh the flask containing the crude product.

10. Extraction of lycopene from tomatoes
Procedure:
1. Weigh 5 g tomato paste in a flask
2. Add 10 ml ethanol and heat for 5 minutes.
3. Filter with filter paper and press to take off all the filtrate
4. Keep the filtrate in conical flask.
5. Put the crude in round-bottom bottle and add 10 ml Dichloromethane, start condensation
6. Boil the solution for 4min. then separate the supernatant and add it to the first filtrate.
7. Repeat this step 3 times.
8. Collect all the filtrate in separating funnel

9. Add 10 ml saturated sodium chloride solution, shake gently and allow separating into 2 layers.

10. Collect the lower layer.

11. Add 1 teaspoon anhydrous sodium sulphate and allow it to stand for 5 minutes.

12. Filter with filter paper.

13. Keep the filtrate in dark bottle away from light otherwise the color of lycopene will disappear.

11. Isolation of Piperine from black pepper
Method:
1. Weigh 50gm of black pepper.
2. Add 300 ml ethanol 95% to the 50 g pepper and hold the condenser above the bottle.
3. Heat the mixture gradually until it is boiled, keep it on heater for 3 hours, then cool it.
4. Filter the mixture in Buchner funnel.
5. Distillate the filtrate in distillation device to remove the extra ethanol until the volume inside reached 25 ml.
6. Then do saponification by adding 25 ml of potassium hydroxide dissolved in ethanol (2 M) to this solvent and then mix it and hold the condenser above the bottle then boil the mixture for exactly 5 min.
7. After this add 35-40 ml water until the solvent become muddy then put it into a beaker then in Ice bath and scratch the wall with a glass rod.

8. Leave it to the next day.
9. Filter the solution in Buchner Funnel.

12. Extraction of Essential Oils from Cinnamon, Clove and *Nigella sativa* by Distillation

Method

1. Weigh 10 g of clove, cinnamon and *Nigella sativa*.
2. Add 100 ml of distilled water and allow standing for 10min with stirring.
3. Start the distillation and collect the distillate. Pour the distillate in separating funnel.
4. Extract the essential oil by 20 ml dichloromethane. Repeat the extraction twice
5. Collect all the extracts in conical flask. Dry with 1spoon anhydrous sodium sulphate, stir for 15 min and then filter in a weighed flask.
6. Evaporate the solvent completely and dry the surface of the conical and weigh the conical again.

13. Extraction of pectin from orange peel and lemon peel

Method

1. The 100-gram dried peels were separately transferred into a beaker (1000 mL) containing 500 mL of water 2.5 mL hydrochloric acid was added to give a pH of 2.2.
2. Each of the fruits was then boiled for 45 min separately.
3. Thereafter, the peels were removed from the extracts by filtering through a filter paper filter study.

4. The cake was washed with 250 mL boiled water and the combined filter allowed to cool to 25°C to minimize heat degradation of the pectin.
5. The extracted pectin was precipitated by adding 200 mL 95% ethanol to 100 mL of the extracted pectin with thorough stirring, left for 30 min to allow the pectin float on the surface.
6. The gelatinous pectin flocculants was then skimmed off.
7. The extracted pectin was purified by washing in 200 mL ethanol and then pressed on a nylon cloth to remove the residual hydrochloric acid and universal salt.
8. The resulting pectin was weighed and shredded into small pieces and was air dried.
9. Finally, the dried pectin was further reduced into smaller pieces using a pestle and mortar and weighed using a digital weighing balance.
10. Percentage yield of pectin from initial wet peels was then determined on both wet and dry weight basis.

14. Isolation of Berberine from *Berberis aristata*
Method
1. Berberine was extracted from powder of *Berberis aristata* roots by Soxhlet apparatus.
2. The ethanolic extract is concentrated on hot water bath till syrupy mass obtained.
3. Dissolve in 25 ml of hot water and filter it with Whatmann filter paper.

4. Add 5 ml hot water to the residual syrupy mass, again filter it.
5. To the combined filtrate add slowly while shaking 15 ml of strong hydrochloric acid (36.5%w/v).
6. Cool it on ice bath for about 30 min or place it in refrigerator for overnight.
7. After cooling filter the contents, wash the crystals of filter paper with water.

15. Extraction of Nicotine from Cigarettes

Procedure:
1. Weigh 10 g of cigarettes leaves in beaker.
2. Add 100 ml of sodium hydroxide solution and stir very well for 15 min.
3. Filter in Buchner using glass wool and press the cigarettes very well by using other beaker.
4. Transfer the cigarettes again to beaker.
5. Add 30 ml distilled water and stir and filter again.
6. Collect the filtrate together. (If there is any impurities re-filter).
7. Transfer the filtrate to the separating funnel and extract by 25 ml ether.
8. Repeat the extraction 3times.
9. Gather the 4 filtrates in conical flask.
10. Dry by using 1teaspoon anhydrous potassium carbonate.
11. Filter and evaporate ether on water bath. (Avoid extra heat because nicotine is hydrolysed by extreme heating).
12. After evaporation of ether add 4 ml methanol to dissolve the resulted oil.

13. Add 10 ml saturated picric acid solution.
14. Cool in an ice bath to precipitate the nicotine di picrate crystals.
15. Filter; allow drying and weighing the product.

16. Extraction of *Lawsonia inermis*

Extraction of Lawsone from the leaf of *Lawsonia inermis* (Henna, Kına):

Method

1. Lawsone occurred in glycosidic form in the leaves. Glycosides have to be cleaved prior study.
2. For this purpose, hydrolysis is required which can be achieved by acidic hydrolysis or keeping in hot water for a long time (24 hr).
3. Dried and powdered leaves contain intact glycosidase which is able to split the glycosidic bond when brought into contact with hot water.
4. Therefore the henna leaf powder suspension is stirred for several hours in hot water at 70°C.
5. Lawsone is not readily soluble in water but acidic.
6. At the end of hydrolysis sodium bicarbonate is added to make the aqueous phase weakly basic (pH 7.5).
7. This process brings lawsone into solution before the suspension is filtered.
8. The filtrate is then acidified and lawsone is extracted into diethyl ether.

9. The colour of lawsone differs from an intense orange-yellow to dark red-brown.

Method II
1. Powder of dried henna leaves (5 g) is placed in a large beaker and distilled water (200 ml) is added together with a magnetic stirring rod.
2. The suspension is stirred on a magnetic stirrer with heating while the temperature is kept at 70°C.
3. After 45 min, the colour of the green suspension turns to brown.
4. After 4 h, solid sodium bicarbonate, (1 g) is added.
5. The suspension is filtered by gravity overnight over three large glass funnels with filter paper (diameter 30 cm). This kind of filtration is slow but works reliably. Attempts to force the pace by suction filtration are not advisable because then colloidal particles will rapidly plug the pores of the filter.
6. The filtrates are combined and acidified to pH 3 by addition of 0.12 M Hydrochloric acid.
7. The brown extract undergoes a clarification in this step and turns slightly cloudy.
8. The swollen plant material is discarded.
9. The filtrate is extracted with diethyl ether (4 x 25 ml).
10. In the final extraction, the ether turns to a very pale yellow, indicating the end of extraction. The aqueous phase does not change its brown colour during extraction but turns clear and can be discarded after the extraction.

11. The combined ethereal phases are washed with water (3 x 10 ml) and dried over Magnesium sulphate.
12. The ether is removed completely in vacuo to leave a reddish brown solid as crude product.

17. Isolation of Hesperidin from Orange Peel Using Soxhlet Extractor

Hesperidin can be isolated by two different methods: -

1. The first method involves extracting the dried citrus peel successively with petroleum ether followed by methanol. The petroleum ether removes the essential oils in the peel and the methanol will extract the glycoside (hesperidin).
2. The second method uses an alkaline extraction of chopped orange peel and acidification of the extract. The hesperidin can then be crystallized from the acidified extract. Because of its highly insoluble, crystalline nature, hesperidin is one of the easiest flavonoids to isolate.

Procedure:

1. 150 mL petroleum ether (40 – 60°C) are filled in a 250 mL round bottom flask with magnetic stir bar.
2. 50g dried and powdered orange peel are placed in the extraction sleeve of a Soxhlet extractor and covered with a little glass wool.

3. A reflux condenser is put on the Soxhlet extraction unit, and then the reaction mixture is stirred and heated for 4 hours under strong reflux.
4. The petroleum ether extract is discarded. In order to remove the adherent petroleum ether, the content of the extraction sleeve is laid out in an extensive crystallization dish.
5. Afterwards the substance is placed again in an extraction sleeve and, like before, but with 150 mL methanol, extracted unless the solvent leaving the extraction sleeve is colourless (1 to 2 hours).
6. The extract is evaporated at the rotary evaporator until syrup consistency is reached. The residue is mixed with 50 mL of 6% acetic acid; the precipitated solid is the crude hesperidine.
7. It is sucked off with a Buchner funnel, washed with 6% acetic acid and dried 60 °C until it is constant in weight.
8. For recrystallization, a 5% solution of the crude product in dimethyl sulfoxide is produced under stirring and heating to 60–80 °C.
9. Afterwards the same amount of water is added slowly whilst stirring.
10. When cooling to room temperature the hesperidine precipitates.
11. It is sucked off, first washed with little warm water and then with isopropanol and dried in the desiccators until it is constant in weight.

TLC-Conditions:

Adsorbant: TLC plates GF254 normal silica

Mobile phase: n-butanol : acetic acid : water = 4 : 1 : 5

Rf (hesperidine) = 0.6

18. Identification of Plant Pigments (Carotenoids) by Thin Layer Chromatography

Procedure:

Developing solvent (mobile phase): 100 mL of petroleum ether, 11 mL of acetone and 5 drops of dist. water Preparation of the TLC chamber: The developing solvent is placed into a TLC chamber. The solvent should completely cover the bottom of the chamber to a depth of approximately 0.5 cm. The chamber is closed and shaken. It is kept covered so that evaporation doesn't change the composition of the developing solvent mixture. After 15 minutes the chamber will be saturated with the solvent vapour.

Extraction of the leaf pigments:

1. Using a pestle fresh leaves are grinded in a mortar containing 22 ml of acetone, 3 ml of petrol ether and a spatula tip-full of calcium carbonate.
2. The pigment extract is filtered.
3. The filtrate is put into a separating funnel and is mixed with 20 ml of petroleum ether and 20 ml of 10% aqueous sodium chloride solution. The separating funnel is shaken carefully.
4. When the layers have separated the lower layer is allowed to drain into a beaker. This phase is thrown away.
5. The upper layer is washed 3-4 times with 5 ml of distilled water.
6. Afterwards the extract is placed in an Erlenmeyer flask and is dried with about 4 spatula tips of sodium sulphate. Filter and

evaporate the solvent on water-bath until the final volume become of about 3 ml.

Application of the extract to the TLC plate:

With a pencil a line is drawn approximately 1.5 cm from the bottom of the plate. The procedure is repeated until the line is very dark green. The transferred extract is allowed to dry thoroughly after each addition. The line is kept as thin and straight as possible.

Experimental procedure:

The loaded TLC plate is carefully placed in the TLC chamber with the sample line toward the bottom. The plate whose top is leaned against the jar wall should sit on the bottom of the chamber and be in contact with the developing solvent (solvent surface must be below the extract line). The TLC chamber is covered. The TLC plate is allowed to remain undisturbed. When the solvent front has reached three quarters of the length of the plate, the plate is removed from the developing chamber and the position of the solvent front is immediately marked.

As the solvent rises by capillary action up through the TLC plate, the components of the pigment mixture are partitioned between the mobile phase (solvent) and the stationary phase (silica gel) due to their different adsorption and solubility strength. The more strongly a given component is adsorbed to the stationary phase, the less easily it is removed by mobile phase. The more weakly a component is adsorbed the faster it will migrate up the TLC plate. On the other hand, the running distance depends on the solubility of the pigment in the solvent. Since the experiment employs a high non-polar solvent (petroleum ether), the pigments that are least polar (carotenes) will be best solved in the non-polar solvent and will thus have the largest running distance.

Rf	leaf pigments	colour
0.95	β-carotenes	golden
0.83	pheophytin	Olive-green
0.65	chlorophyll a	blue green
0.45	chlorophyll b	yellow green
0.71	xanthophyll	Yellow-brown

19. TLC Analysis of Curcumin and its Derivatives of Turmeric

Preparation of Extract *Curcuma longa* (Zingiberaceae), Turmeric

Powdered drug (1 g) is extracted with methylene chloride (= Dichloromethane, 10 mL) using homogenizator at room temperature for 5 min. The clear filtrate is used for TLC.

Thin-Layer Chromatography (TLC)

Reference solution: A mixture of curcuminoids are dissolved in 1 mL methanol and is used for TLC investigation.

Adsorbent: Silica gel 60 F_{254} precoated TLC plates

Solvent system: Methylene chloride-Methanol (99:1)

Rf of Curcumin: 0.45

Rf of Demethoxycurcumin: 0.20

Rf of BisdemethoxyCurcumin: 0.08

Detection

a. All curcuminoids show quenching in UV-254 nm.

b. All curcuminoids are observed as yellow spots on TLC plate in day light.

c. All curcuminoids show pale yellow fluorescence in UV-365 nm.

20. Thin Layer Chromatography (TLC) of flavonoid drugs
Flavonoid containing Herbal Drugs:

Families	Drugs	Plants	Main flavonoids
Asteraceae	Arnicae flos	*Arnica montana*	Quercetin glycosides
	Anthemidis flos	*Anthemis nobilis* (syn: *Chamaemelum nobile*)	Apigenin and luteolin glycosides
	Calendula flos	*Calendula officinalis*	Isorhamnetin and Quercetin glycosides
	Farfarae flos	*Tussilago farfara*	Quercetin glycosides
	Matricaria flos	*Chamomilla recutita*	Quercimeritrin, apigenin, luteolin, patuletin glycosides.
	Cardui mariae fructus	*Silybum marianum*	Flavonolignans : Silybin, silychristin, silydianin

Primulaceae	Primula flos	*Primula veris, P. elatior*	Quercetin and Gossypetin glycoside
Rosaceae	Crataegi flos	*Crataegus monogyna C. pentagyna, C. nigra, C. azarolus*	Quercetin, apigenin glycosides, flavon C-glycoside(vitexin)
Caprifoliaceae	Sambuci flos	*Sambucus nigra*	Quercetin glycosides
Tiliaceae	Tilia flos	*Tilia cordata*	Quercetin, kaempferol and myrcetin glycosides
Scrophulariaceae	Verbasci flos	*Verbascum phlomoides V. thapsiforma*	Flavonol-glycosides Rutin, hesperidin
Betulaceae	Betulae folium	*Betula pendula, B. pubescens*	Quercetin and myrcetin glycosides
Juglandaceae	Juglandis folium	*Juglans regia*	Hyperoside
Rutaceae	Aurantii pericarpium	*Citrus aurantium ssp. aurantium*	Eriocitrin, rutin Naringenin, naringin, hesperidin, neohesperidin, sinensetin

Rutaceae	Citri pericarpium	*Citrus medis*	Eriocitrin, rutin, Neohesperidin, naringenin 7-O-hesperidoside
Lamiaceae	Orthosiphonus folium	*Orthosiphon spicatus*	Flavonoid aglycones: Sinensetin (pentamethoxy flavon), scutellareintetr amethylether, eupatorin

Preparation of drug extracts for TLC:

Drugs: One of the drugs listed above. Pulver drugs (each 1 g) is extracted in 10 ml methanol at 60° C for 5 minutes by keeping in ultrasonic bath. The filtrate is concentrated to a few ml, of which 20 µl is applied on to the TLC.

Exceptions:

Cardui mariae fructus (*Slybi fructus*): 1 g Pulver drug is extracted first with 50 ml petroleum ether under reflux to remove lipophillic compounds. The defatted drug is further extracted with 10 ml methanol for 10 min. The filtrate is concentrated to 5 ml, of which 30 µl is applied on to the TLC.

Farfara folium, Petasites folium: Pulver drug (each 2 g) is extracted with 10 ml dichloromethane for 15 min under reflux. The filtrate is concentrated to a few ml, of which 20 µl is applied on to the TLC. Reference solution: Each of the available reference compounds is dissolved in methanol (0.05%). At least 10 µl of the reference solution should be applied on TLC plate.

Adsorbent: TLC Silica gel 60 F_{254}

Mobile phase (Solvent system):

1. Ethylacetate – Formic acid – Acetic acid – Water (100:11:11:27)
2. Ethylacetate – Acetic acid – Water (66:15:20)
3. Ethylacetate – Formic acid – Acetic acid – Ethylmethylketone-Water (50:7:3:30:10)
4. Chloroform – Aceton – Formic acid (75:16.5:8.5)
5. Chloroform – Ethylacetate (60:40)
6. n-Butanol – Acetic acid – Water (40:10:50; upper phase) (For cellulose plates)

Detection:

Direct evaluation:

UV254: All flavonoids give a fluorescence reduction in form of dark-blue zones on yellow background of the plates.

UV365: According to their structure types, flavonoids represent yellow, blue or green fluorescence.

Spraying reagents

Modified Naturstoff–Reagent:1% Diphenylboryloxy ethyl-amine solution in methanol. After spraying, immediately and/or after 15 min, typical intensive fluorescence colors in the UV 365 nm are developed. The additive of PEG (Polyethylene glycol) leads also to an increase of the detection limit (from 10 µg to 0,5 µg). The fluorescence behavior is structural-dependent.

i. Flavonols: Quercetin and myrcetin glycosides give orange

ii. Kaemferol and isorhamnetin glycosides give yellowish green

iii. Flavons: Luteolin glycosides give orange colours while apigenin glycosides yellowish green.

21. Thin Layer Chromatography (TLC) of Anthocyanins and Crocin

Anthocyanin and Crocin containing Herbal Drugs

Families	Drugs	Plants	Main flavonoids
Asteraceae	Cyani flos	*Centaurea cyanus*	Cyanin and pelargonidin glycosides
Malvaceae	Hibisci flos	*Hibiscus sabdariffa*	Hibiscin (Delphinidin glycoside)
	Malvae flos	*Malva sylvestris*	Malvin (Malvidin diglucoside)
	Malvae (arboreae) flos	*Althaea rosea*	Delphinidin and malvidin glucosides

Crocin and adulteration (False saffron)			
Iridaceae	Croci stigma	*Crocus sativa*	Crocin, picrocrocin
Asteraceae	Carthamus flos	*Carthamus tinctoria*	

Extraction and characterization

Anthocyanins are soluble in water and alcohols, and insoluble in apolar organic solvents. They are generally extracted with an alcohol (Methanol, Ethanol) in the presence of a small amount (0.1 – 1%) of hydrochloric acid. To avoid esterification of the free carboxyl group of acylated anthocyanins by a diacid, and especially to prevent their deacylation, it is beter to use other acids (acetic acid, tartaric acid), and to work at low temperature. Anthocyanin solutions are very unstable, and they can only be kept under nitrogen, at low temperature, and in the dark.

Preparation of drug extracts for TLC:

Drugs are listed above.

Anthocyanin drugs: Pulver drugs (each 1 g) is extracted with 6 ml a mixture of Methanol and 25% HCl (9:1) for 10 minutes by keeping in ultrasonic bath. After filtration, 25 µl is applied on to the TLC. Croci stigma: 4 – 5 dried *Crocus sativus* stigma are moistened with water: After 3 min 1 ml Methanol is added and extracted by shaking for 10 min in dark. It can be directly applied on to TLC plate. Reference solution: Anthocyanins (each 1 mg) is dissolved in 1 ml Methanol. At least 5 µl is applied on TLC plate.

Methylene blue: 5 mg is dissolved in 10 ml Methanol.

Naphtol yellow: 5 mg is dissolved in 5 ml Methanol.

Sudan red: 5 mg is dissolved in 10 ml Methanol.

Adsorbent: TLC Silica gel 60 F_{254} TLC Cellulose

Mobile phase (Solvent system):

Anthocyanins: n-Butanol – Acetic acid – Water (40:10:20) (For cellulose and Silica gel plates)

Croci stigma: Ethylacetate – isopropanol – Water (65:25:10)

Detection:

1. Direct evaluation: Anthocyanins give visible red to blue – violet colours.
2. Compounds of Croci stigma give yellow colours.

22. Identification of Anthraquinone Glycosides from Plant Extract

I. Extraction of the free anthraquinone:

1. In a test tube add 10 ml Petroleum ether to 2 gm of powdered drug.

2. Shake for 10 minutes and filter through a filter paper into a test tube and keep marc on the filter paper, spot the filtrate on TLC plate.

3. Add 5 ml of the standard alkali (potassium hydroxide or 10% ammonia).

4. Observe and record the colour which develops immediately or upon standing for a few minutes.

II. Extraction of the anthraquinone glycoside:

5. Transfer the marc on the filter paper in step 2 into conical flask or a beaker and add to it 20 ml of 50% ethanol.

6. Boil for 5 minutes on a water bath.

7. Filter while warm through cotton wool into graduated beaker, spot the filtrate into the TLC plate then wash with hot alcohol to adjust the volume to 20 ml.

III. Testing for anthraquinone O- glycoside

8. Transfer 10 ml of the glycosidic extract powder produced in step 7 into a conical flask or a beaker and add to it 10 ml of 25% Hydrochloric acid.

9. Boil for 15 minutes over a boiling water bath.

10. Cool the solution and transfer into a separating funnel.

11. Shake the solution with 10 ml petroleum ether in the separating funnel.

12. Separate the organic layer into a test tube, spot the petroleum ether extract onto the TLC plate then shake the organic layer with 5 ml of the standard alkali.

13. Observe and record the colour produced on standing for few minutes and observe any change in colour

IV. Testing for the anthraquinone C- Glycosides:

14. Transfer 10 ml of the glycoside extract produced in step 7 into a conical flask and adds 1 g of Ferric chloride and heat for 20 minutes on a boiling water bath.

15. Cool the solution down and then transfer into a separating funnel.

16. Extract the solution with 10 ml chloroform and separate the aqueous layer from the chloroform layer.

17. Wash the organic layer with water and transfer the chloroform layer into a test tube, spot the organic layer onto the TLC plate.

18. Add 5 ml of the standard alkali then observe and record the colour formed immediately and on standing for a few minutes.

V. Thin layer chromatography:

19. Develop the TLC on the mobile phase

20. Examine the plate under day and both long and short UV lights

21. Spray the plate with alcoholic potassium hydroxide spraying reagent.

22. Heat the plate for 10 minutes to intensify the colours and examine the chromatogram under the day and UV lights.

References:

1. Wagner, H, Bladt, S, Zgainski, E.M. Drogen analyse: DC Analyse von Arzneidrogen, Springer-Verlag, Berlin, 1983.
2. CLASSICS IN SPECTROSCOPY – Isolation and Structure Elucidation of Natural Products, Stefan BERGER & Dieter SICKER, WILEY-VCH, Weinheim, 2009.
3. Fieser L.F and Williamson, K.L. Organic Experiments, 6/e, D. C. Heath and Co., Lexington, MA, 1987.
4. Pavia, D.L, Lampman, G.M, Kriz, G.S, Engel, R.G. Introduction to Organic Laboratory Techniques, A Microscale Approach, Saunders College Publications, San Francisco, 1990.

5. Pavia, D.L., Lampman, G.M. and Kriz, G.S. Introduction to organic laboratory technique, W. B. Saunders Co., Philadelphia, 1976, p. 50-54.
6. Britton, G. Structure and properties of carotenoids in relation to function. FASEB J., 1995, 9:15511558.
7. Britton, G.S. Liaaen-Jensen and Pfander, H. Carotenoids today and challenges for the future. In: Britton, G, Liaaen-Jensen, S and Pfander H. [eds], Carotenoids vol. 1A: Isolation and Analysis. Basel: Birkh user, 1995.
8. Mercadante, A. New carotenoids: recent progress. Invited Lecture 2. Abstracts of the 12th International Carotenoid Symposium, Cairns, Australia, July 1999.
9. Ong, A.S.H., and E.S. Tee. Natural sources of carotenoids from plants and oils. Meth. Enzymol., 1992, 213: 142-167.
10. Pfander, H. Carotenoids: an overview. Meth. Enzymol., 1992, 213: 3-13.
11. Mimansha, C.P. Isolation of Berberine from *Berberis aristata* by an Acid Dye Method and Optimization of Parameters, International Journal of Pharmaceutical Sciences Review and Research, 20(2), 2013, 34: 187-189

www.ingramcontent.com/pod-product-compliance
Lightning Source LLC
Chambersburg PA
CBHW050242230526
45470CB00005B/2079